BEING BEAR

BEING BEAR

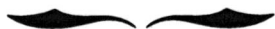

JOY PERSHING

authorHOUSE®

AuthorHouse™
1663 Liberty Drive
Bloomington, IN 47403
www.authorhouse.com
Phone: 1-800-839-8640

Published by AuthorHouse   10/18/2012

ISBN: 978-1-4772-5855-2 (sc)
ISBN: 978-1-4772-7446-0 (e)

Library of Congress Control Number: 2012917827

Any people depicted in stock imagery provided by Thinkstock are models, and such images are being used for illustrative purposes only. Certain stock imagery © Thinkstock.

This book is printed on acid-free paper.

CONTENTS

INTRODUCTION

"Every good and perfect gift is from above."
—James 1:17

Growing up with an older brother who was diagnosed with Down's syndrome was as normal to me as Christmas trees in December. As the youngest of seven children, I never knew life to be any different. Truthfully, my brother Paul never seemed less "normal" than any of my other five brothers pounding through the house. As I grew older and began to realize how special Paul was, I remember thinking that *we* were the lucky ones—the chosen ones who were fortunate enough to have a brother like him. As adults, we still feel the same way.

Paul was born fourth of seven children. Dave, Steve, and Mark came before him and Tim, Matt, and me, Joy, followed after. We were all born and raised in Greencastle, Indiana, by our parents, Jerry and Marcia Tesmer. Six boys, one girl! Our family has since expanded to more than twenty-six, including sisters-in-law (Carla, Cathy, Kim, Crystal), one brother-in-law (Brian), and ten grandchildren (Jerry, Andrew, Ashley, Katie, Brandon, Braden, Noah, Arianna, Emeline, and Thomas).

Paul has always had a knack for bringing the very best out in people. It wasn't until the death of our second sibling, Steve, that I felt the need to write a book about the impact Paul has had on this world while we are still blessed to have him here. Reality hit home on February 16, 2010 when Steve joined our Heavenly Father, who took with him the countless, undocumented stories and memories of this most exceptional human being, Paul Samuel Tesmer. It is in honor of Paul and my parents and in memory of Steve that I write about Paul's life.

CHAPTER ONE

A Life Worth Saving

"If anyone does not provide for his
relatives, and especially for his immediate
family, he has denied the faith and is worse
than an unbeliever."
—1 Timothy 5:8

Imagine waiting nine months to meet the miracle growing inside of you, only to experience the doctors and nurses immediately taking the baby into isolation and away from his mother. On May 28, 1969, this was the case for my then twenty-four-year-old mother. During the late sixties our county hospital placed multiple expectant mothers in a labor room until they were ready to deliver their babies; privacy was not regularly afforded as it is today.

While the other mothers were cooing and ahhing at their new baby bundles, my mother was panicking and praying for God to help save the tiny new life she brought into the world. Having had three children, she was well practiced on the process of babies and birthing and knew instantly that something was not right.

At her first glimpse, Mom knew that Paul looked different than her preceding newborns. His eyes were significantly almond shaped and his hands and fingers appeared unusually small. Her assumption was confirmed when the doctors told her they wanted to send Paul to Indianapolis to conduct further tests.

Paul was the first baby with Down's syndrome that my mother's doctor had ever delivered. He delivered the grim news to Dad in the isolation room. After explaining to my father that he thought Paul might have a condition called Down's syndrome, Dr. Fred Haggerty picked up Paul and showed Dad that a healthy newborn should stiffen their limbs if they were not held securely. As Dad witnessed, Paul's limbs were naturally relaxed in the doctor's open hands. It was Dr. Haggerty that suggested that Dad and Mom take Paul to a larger hospital in Indianapolis, where they would be better equipped to handle cases like this.

Mom left the hospital the same day that she delivered Paul, which was uncharacteristic in 1969, when most postpartum hospital stays were three days. However, inside she felt a new fire to save the life that God had entrusted to her and she did not want to waste one second. Paul was born with a compromised immune system and the sooner he could get access to more advanced care, the better his future outlook would be.

Mom and Dad wanted Dave, Steve, and Mark to meet their new brother, so before making the hour-long journey to Indianapolis, the three boys smiled at him through a car window, welcoming the new baby into their world. Mom remembers how Steve was instantly drawn to Paul; that bond proved to last a lifetime and beyond. Dad explained to the siblings that Paul needed to see some special doctors in Indianapolis and that he, Mom, and the baby would be back home soon.

Riley Children's Hospital confirmed Dr. Haggerty's original hypothesis that Paul was born with Down's syndrome and that he was at the "severely profound" level on the spectrum of mental retardation. The doctors at Riley carefully explained that Paul's sucking reflex was not functioning and that they were unable to get him to drink milk or medicine on his own. Dad remembers watching Paul's infant body turn tragically lethargic, and Mom remembers that with each passing hour, Paul's body became more and more lifeless. My parents were encouraged to leave him at the hospital where, if he survived, he would be placed in a special facility with other children with conditions as severe as his, and he would receive immediate and cutting-edge medical treatment. Dad remembers being advised that leaving Paul in institutional care was in the best interest of their other three children as well. The chances of long term survival for Paul at that time were slim, according to the statistics presented to them. After experiencing all the wonderful times we have had with Paul, the idea of leaving him with an institution seems appalling, however, our family has always credited Riley Children's Hospital for being open and honest with their advice. Furthermore, their comprehensive and aggressive care has saved Paul's life many times.

My parents *never* take the easy way out. They are strong, conservative Christians, and their faith and trust in God is what led them to do what others might have classified as insane. Dad checked Paul out of the hospital and brought him home, and Mom diligently worked with Paul to develop a sucking reflex so they could nourish his already-struggling body. Mom recalls that during the day Paul remained lifeless, but she continued to try to breastfeed him. She remembers the moment that his sucking reflex started working, because he did not want to stop eating once he started. As she recalls the moment, she smiles with pride that in a short time, he was sporting quite the baby belly!

Paul was doing well nursing and did not start having problems until he was almost one year old. He immediately started getting sick after he was weaned. Over the next three and a half years, Paul was in the hospital more than he was at home. His health did not improve until they met with Dr. Brown, an immune specialist, who sent Paul to Methodist Hospital in Indianapolis to begin a series of shots that would boost his immune system. Mom and Dad drove Paul to Indianapolis daily for the injections; Paul's health improved significantly with each shot. Eventually, Dr. Haggerty was able to start giving the shots to Paul in Greencastle.

Paul continues to battle pneumonia, ear infections, sinus infections, eye infections, asthma, allergies, arthritis, and dental issues forty-two years later. These illnesses are compounded by the fact that my parents have to keep a watchful eye on him at all times because of his inability to communicate exactly what is hurting him. Paul is not one to complain, and early detection through Mom and Dad's finely-honed insight, is key to his survival. However, Paul doesn't let their concern get him down or set him back. He asks for prayer and believes that God will answer him. And, God answers!

CHAPTER TWO

Growing Up Normal with a "Dis"ability

*"I can do everything through him who
gives me strength."*
—Philippians 4:13

Dad recalls the conversation he had with Mom when they concluded that God had an earthly purpose for Paul to fulfill, and that all attempts should be made to treat him like the rest of their children. This meant placing the least amount of restrictions on him so he could grow and learn as an individual, while still maintaining his health and safety. They had normalized him so much that it wasn't until I was five years old and Paul was ten that I learned he had been born with a disability.

ONE SUMMER'S DAY

I remember most everything about the steamy summer afternoon when I found some loose change around our house and asked Mom if I could use it to buy a piece of candy at the candy store. She agreed, as long as I took one of my brothers with me. I interrupted Matt and Tim playing in the back yard to see if they would take me, and they both said no; so I asked Paul. I remember looking up at him with full faith that he would and could take me, and he obligingly agreed. He helped me into our little red wagon and he pulled me the three blocks to the corner grocery store just off of the DePauw University campus.

Once inside, Paul quickly found his favorite candy—Sixlets chocolates. As I was perusing the bounty of sweets for my final selection, Mom and some of our brothers stampeded through the grocery doors in a surprising panic. I began to cry at all of the fuss around me; I didn't understand why Mom was so distressed. I knew for sure that she agreed to let me go as long as I took one of my brothers!

It was later that day when she explained to me the hazard in taking Paul out alone, since people in the community would not likely be able to understand his speech or unique sign language like we could. She continued to clarify that if he and I were to get lost, Paul would not be able to explain who he was or where we lived. I remember curiously wondering how any cogent person would have difficulty communicating with him.

I started to understand more clearly that summer Mom's concern regarding Paul's lack of ability to communicate with others when he started to sneak away on his own. Paul became very familiar with the DePauw campus, including the various dormitories and fraternity and sorority houses. DePauw became quite comfortable with him as well. Mom did not like us to watch TV after our morning cartoons and Paul understood clearly that the fraternity and sorority houses had several television sets. It was not uncommon for a student to walk into their room and find Paul sitting on their bed watching their TV. It didn't take long until they had our phone number posted by their telephones to report that Paul had slipped away again.

THE RUNAWAY

Paul continued his endeavor as a runaway in other various areas of life. For instance, with seven children in the house, Mom delegated summer chores to everyone, including Paul. It was understood that while Mom cleaned or cooked for us inside the house, we were responsible for helping watch Paul. This duty fell more on the boys than me, since I rarely left Mom's side. Paul was known at the time for being an escape artist—even better than Houdini himself! Paul could back away from you right in front of your own eyes and you would never notice him running off. The police often helped us find him as we would try to recreate his invisible path. Paul learned to be so quiet that you could walk right past him without knowing it; he was as quiet as a mouse and as still as a deer.

One time my parents took us to the Indianapolis Museum of Art; Dad recalls holding Paul's hand through the museum, while showing Paul an exhibit. When he looked down at Paul, he realized he was holding another child's hand! Paul took a random child and quietly placed his hand in Dad's hand, allowing him to sneak away . . . again. We also frequented the Indianapolis Children's Museum. We had to be especially cautious at this museum because Paul always wants to ride the carousel on the top floor; he made several attempts over the years to casually break away from the family and go back to the carousel.

VANISHING FOOD TRAP

Paul was also known for another subtle move that we called the vanishing food trap. We were expected to eat everything Mom put on our plates during meal time, and we were to waste nothing. Mom's rule was that even if you don't like it, you still have to try it. As you can imagine feeding nine people at one time caused Mom to run frequently from our dining room table to the kitchen, while Dad's routine was to help Mom tidy the kitchen as we finished off the vegetables that we didn't like.

Our kitchen had a swinging door separating it from the dining room. When Mom and Dad would depart into the kitchen and the door would swing shut, the Vanishing Food Trap process would begin. Whoever didn't want to eat something unpleasant on their plate would quietly say to Paul in Step One, "Do not touch my plate, and do not eat my food." Step Two was to walk away from the table. This was followed by Step Three, where Paul would hastily rush to the plate and consume every last crumb. Step Four was to walk back in to the dining room and pretend like you were upset that he ate your food.

Since the family rule was to sit at the table until you cleaned your plate, Paul made it very easy for the rest of us to get to Step Five, which was to move along with our evening. This worked flawlessly until Mom and Dad became aware of our deceptive arrangement.

THE WRESTLING DAYS

Paul became fascinated with wrestling around the age of ten, and soon Saturday mornings in the Tesmer house gave way to WWF wrestling matches with the likes of the great Hulk Hogan, the Sheik, and Paul's all-time favorite, Dick the Bruiser. As the youngest child and the only girl besides Mom in the house, I resented the power that wrestling had over Paul because he was in no way partial when it came to picking out his next wrestling opponent!

Dave, the oldest sibling, fueled Paul's passion for the sport. Dave taught Paul all of the different moves and holds before they would stage different jumps and stunts where Paul would end up flipping Dave over his back. During this phase of Paul's life, we quickly and sometimes painfully discovered that it was no longer safe to lie on the floor to watch TV, or we would risk an elbow or knee drop followed by a headlock from a very animated boy-wrestler!

Tim, the fifth youngest sibling, recalls how Paul loved to put him and Matt in a headlock. They would lean forward at the waist as Paul would hit them on the back with a synchronized foot stomp, as seen on Saturday-morning wrestling. This stomp was to make the hit on the back sound significantly harder than it really was. While the boys have a fondness with the wrestling days, I was happy when he moved on to something else! Wrestling was not my idea of fun role-playing.

Matt and Tim, brothers number five and six, remember Paul jumping off of the back of the couch onto whichever one of them was ready and awaiting a new match. Paul also cherished the role as the announcer; he would assert in an exceptionally stadium-like voice, as clearly as he possibly could, "In this corner weighing in at seventy-five pounds, from Greencastle, Indiana . . . Matthew Robert." He would raise Matt's arm and move over to Tim and announce him the same way. Paul loved to watch them wrestle as much as he loved to put people in different wrestling holds. The only drawback that my brothers could recall during this time was that that he would not let them win against him or even wrestle him back. If any of the boys put him in a playful wrestling hold he would cry out, "Mommy!" or, "Daddy!"

Tim recalls how Paul used to be the first person to run out the doors of our church on Sunday evenings so he could strategically place himself to await his weekly victim, our cousin Joe, and inflict his perfected headlock on him. Joe knew this was coming every Sunday night, but always pretended to be surprised when Paul would jump out and wrangle him into a hold.

BOY SCOUTS

Dad became a Boy Scout leader when our oldest brother Dave was old enough to join. Dad spent many years taking his sons and their troop members to camps and pinewood derbies. As soon as they were eligible, Steve, Mark, and Paul joined the group, too. When Paul became a Boy Scout, he loved wearing his brown uniform and scarf and attending the meetings with Dad as his leader.

Paul participated in the activities alongside his scout mates and truly loved spending time outside. Paul and Dad attended a camp at Bradford Woods near Bloomington, Indiana one year, and they got turned around in the woods, which led to several miles and hours of hiking. It was dark when they finally made their way back to their cabin. Unfortunately, they forgot to bring their sleeping bags from the car. After spending the night covering up in some plastic that they found in the closet of the cabin, Paul missed the comforts of home. When the camp was finally over, so were his Boy Scout days; he told Dad he was finished.

FAVORITE TELEVISION SHOWS

As a young boy, Paul was mesmerized with the TV shows *Batman*, *The Dukes of Hazard* (Boss Hog was his favorite character), *The Incredible Hulk*, and *The A-Team* (B. A. Baracus was the man!). We were not allowed to turn the television on during the day, so in the late afternoon when we were able to watch it, Paul turned on his shows and we all watched with him. None of the other siblings thought it was unfair that he picked out the shows, we were happy enough just to watch TV.

During the fighting scenes Paul would jump up to join in the on-screen fight by air-punching the "bad guys," who were invisible to the rest of us, but very real to him. He made sounds with his mouth like "PSHHHH, PSHHH, PSHHH" with every punch as he desperately helped Batman and Robin defeat the Joker or other super-villains.

WHAT'S NORMAL?

If being a normal kid means loving superheroes, watching television, loving sports, swimming, and eating, then my parents' goal of establishing normalcy in Paul's life was realized. Paul could drive up and down the road in front of our house on his big, bad, pedal-powered, three-wheeled, Green Machine faster than any kid on the block! He was able to make life-long friends that he still holds dearly and works with even today. Mom and Dad found a way of minimizing the "dis" and maximizing the "ability" in Paul's disability.

CHAPTER THREE

Santa Is for Real

"Each of you should look not only to your own interests, but also to the interests of others."
—Philippians 2:4

Christmas in the Tesmer household is the most extraordinary time of the year! It isn't purely the gifts that bring enchantment to the season, though they are certainly an added bonus. It is the magic that Paul displays in his belief in Santa Clause as well as his affection for the Douglass-fir evergreen Christmas tree.

For over thirty years, Paul, by tradition, has requested Santa to bring him a Beach Boys cassette tape. He has numerous copies of Beach Boys albums in a variety of musical formats, including records, cassette tapes, and CD's. But Christmas just isn't Christmas without opening something Beach Boys or Coca Cola related under the tree on Christmas morning. Traditionally Paul sits on Santa's lap each year at the same mall and, as of the past few Christmases, Santa (a friend of the family donning a bright red suit and beard) has shown up at my house delivering Paul presents under our tree before Christmas. Santa, our friend, will also call Paul around his birthday each year or if he is sick in the hospital.

THE BIG HUNT

Our family is firmly rooted in traditions, and since he was a child, the most anticipated tradition was the quest for the perfect Christmas tree! Every year Paul reminds family members, friends, and strangers, at least four to six months in advance, that he wants to look for a Christmas tree. Long ago, Paul made up his own hand signal for a Christmas tree with twinkling lights. While we made the voyage only once a year, Paul can still tell you which way to turn and how to get to the only place in the world one would ever want to buy a Christmas tree, Wagoner Christmas Tree Farm, just north of Greencastle.

We almost always went on a Sunday in December, right after church. I remember well into adulthood the tradition of going to church, eating lunch, and driving the nearly twenty-mile journey to the middle of nowhere for the perfect tree. As we would round the final turn of the long driveway, heading up a small hill, the image of the country Christmas tree farm was captivating. It looked like miles and miles of evergreens cast into infinity; some trees stood straight, tall, and powerful, while others were barren, tilted, and small. The weather was never a factor for any of us. We have picked out trees in rain, snow, sleet, and ice, only adding to the thrill of our quest. Unfortunately today due to allergies, Paul cannot have a real Christmas tree in his house. However, he still gets to make the voyage to help our third-oldest brother, Mark, pick out a tree with his family.

When arriving at the Christmas tree farm, Paul would always be the first to jump out of the car the moment it stopped. He would run into the office to pick up the coveted orange handsaw that the tree farm provided. It was understood that Paul was in charge of cutting the tree down, and his siblings simply knew not to suggest a turn for someone else. None of us would have wanted to anyway; it was too much fun watching him climb under the tree with the focus of a surgeon. The jokesters in our family always took the saw away from Paul, found the puniest tree around, and pretended that they were going to cut it down and bring it home. Paul would pout, tell Mom and Dad that he didn't want that tree, and they would reassure him that we were only teasing him. I guess it was so much fun to hear his cries of displeasure as he would, with very little energy, moan "Ughhhh-huuuuu" to Mom and Dad, to signify that he didn't want to joke around about such an important issue.

This was Paul's big hunt, and the thrill was that we always knew that he would pick a twelve to twenty foot tall tree; Mom and Dad would have to always suggest that he find a smaller tree that would fit into our house. Not one time did he fail us in picking out an extra large Christmas tree! In his mind, the perfect tree is around twelve feet tall, deep green in color, lacking any barren spots, and has a branch-spread of at least eight feet. Realistically, he had to settle with a seven to eight foot tree that would later be trimmed to fit into our living room.

CHRISTMAS IN FLORIDA?

Paul is stubborn; and he is set in his ways, which are based on traditions of doing things the same way year after year. This was confirmed the year that we spent Christmas in Florida instead of Indiana. We moved to Florida for six months for business purposes while Dad worked on a building project in Fort Myers. We rented a house in Punta Gorda. Paul loved the sun and water, but he did not understand why it was so warm during the holiday season. That Christmas, Paul was invited to ride on a float in the local Christmas parade and Mom remembers how horrified he was to see Santa Claus riding in a float on a hot steamy day, baring his chest from an unbuttoned red Santa suit!

Another issue Paul had with that sunny Christmas season, besides the warm temperatures, was there was no nearby Christmas tree farm with a bright-orange handsaw to cut and trim your own tree. Paul was not happy the evening our parents took us to the grocery store to buy a Boy Scout Christmas tree, which was leaning up against the storefront. Paul was so miserable with the selection that he did not want to help decorate the tree with our time-honored decorations. In fact, he did not want it to be decorated at all.

Christmas day that year was warm enough to go to the ocean and swim. It was so much fun for the rest of the family to swim outside in December, except for Paul. He was completely discontented and perplexed that it was so hot outside on Christmas.

When we got home from the beach that Christmas afternoon and were changing into dry clothes, Paul quietly walked into the family room where the Christmas tree was located. He opened the front door, and dragged the entire Christmas tree, garland and all, onto the front lawn. To Paul, Christmas was not about swimming in the ocean or Santa Claus baring his chest. It was about making the journey to Wagoner Christmas Tree Farm, white snow, bright-orange handsaws, and a fully dressed Santa.

A Resourceful Christmas!

The following Christmas we were at last back in Indiana but we were living in Plainfield, which is about a fifty-minute drive from Wagoner Christmas Tree Farm. So, yet again, we found ourselves resorting to a local grocery store with Boy Scout Christmas trees leaning up against the side.

That particular Christmas we were financially-strapped and had to settle on a small, inexpensive, but real tree. For the second year in a row Paul was not happy about the circumstances, and he had little difficulty in rejecting the tree and finding a resourceful solution to his Christmas dilemma.

Our neighbor to the north of us had a beautiful evergreen tree that stood arrogantly around nine feet tall, and just as wide. One day after bringing home the store-bought Christmas tree, Paul practiced his escape artists' techniques. He quietly ventured out to the garage and found dad's handsaw. He proceeded to walk over to the house next door, and discreetly cut down the attractive tree, leaving an exposed and naked blemish around our neighbor's front porch. We were blessed at the time to have accepting and considerate neighbors.

THE EXPLANATION

Paul understood from many years of our family traditions that the Christmas season is truly about the birth of our savior, Jesus Christ. However, Paul loved Santa Claus so much that he would not believe that Santa was not real. To imply such an insensitive thought would make him cry and tattle on us to Mom. He would not accept that Santa was our dad, and after several failed attempts at trying to explain the concept of Santa Claus, it was easier to join instead of dispute him.

SANTA'S DIAL-A-PRAYER

Because of Paul's insistence on Santa's existence, Santa became very real to each person in our family. During the late eighties and early nineties a local church opened a phone line called Dial-A-Prayer, so that anyone could call in and hear a short Bible verse followed by a pre-recorded prayer for that day. It is unclear who thought that Paul would enjoy the pre-recorded phone devotion, but someone in our family dialed the number for Paul, and he became obsessed with the telephone from that point on.

Paul was convinced that the Reverend Paul Bowen, whose Australian voice could be heard on Dial-A-Prayer, was in fact Santa Claus trying to spread God's Word. Paul could not remember all of the numbers to dial, so someone always needed to dial the number for him, but once the number was in, he would hang up and hit the redial button to listen to that day's prayer again and again.

Redialing posed several challenges for me that, as a high school student, nearly drove me to insanity. First off, if I was at track or cross country practice and needed to call Mom to ask her to pick me up earlier or later, I could never get through. Paul was continually hanging up and redialing to hear Santa's message and it would tie up the phone line. Next, we only had one phone at our house and if Paul was using it, I couldn't socialize with my friends or call my boyfriend, who was eventually my husband, Brian. Fighting Paul over the phone was maddening because he was just as stubborn as I, and neither of us would budge on whose turn it was to have possession over the phone. I finally got smart and resorted to his tactics of telling Mom so she would make him give me a turn on the phone.

For Dad, Paul tying up the phone line was an economical issue since he relied on clients to call him at home for construction and building jobs. It seemed that the more Mom tried to monitor Paul calling Santa on Dial-A-Prayer, the more obsessed he became about calling it. We always had to remember that if we dialed a number out to redial Santa's number, or he would push the redial button and dial the last number called.

THE PRANK CALLER

My husband Brian recalls a time when I called him and we talked for over an hour on the phone. After we ended our call, my head was apparently in the clouds as I walked up to my bedroom to get ready for bed and completely forgot to redial Santa's number. Paul waited patiently for my departure before he picked up the phone and hit redial. When

Brian's dad, Gary, answered their home phone he heard only silence on the other end. As soon as Gary would hang up the phone, it would immediately ring again. Brian's patient father was getting frustrated at the prank caller and after five or six prank calls, Gary started yelling into the phone. Immediately Brian put two and two together, and answered the phone on the next ring. After saying, "Hello," and hearing nothing, Brian said, "Hi, Paul!" A surprised Paul responded "Hi, Bri (which he pronounces 'Nih')!" And alas the mystery of the prank caller was solved.

SANTA'S HOME

Another feature of Santa's life that Paul invented was where Santa and his reindeer live. For reasons we may never know, Paul selected an old, dilapidated trailer home near Highway 40 as the official home of Santa Claus. As we would approach that part of the road, Paul could hardly contain his excitement at passing Santa's house.

He would begin shouting to Santa Claus (which he pronounced Kubba-Kaws), "Hi, Santa Claus! Hi, Santa Claus! Hi, Santa Claus! Hi, Santa Claus!" He would continue his mantra until we were well away from the beloved site of worship. It was very charming and engaging when he first started doing it, but there was nothing more irritating on a return trip from Indianapolis, late at night, with everyone snuggled quietly in the car, than being suddenly awakened by Paul's intense shouting. Although the trailer has been removed from the site, Paul can still be heard telling Santa hello—thankfully his greeting is less emphatic now.

BEAUTY IS IN THE EYE OF THE BEHOLDER

Does something have to be tangible in order for it to be real? Christians do not think so. We believe in God, who sent us His Son, who we have not seen either, but believe in very much. A Christian would not dispute God's existence on the grounds of the unseen. This is why Santa is real to those of us around Paul. It is his genuine belief in Santa Claus that has magically transformed Christmas, adding to the beauty of the season.

Chapter Four

Heaven, Praying, Church, and Dying

*"The prayer of a righteous man is powerful
and effective."*
—James 5:16

Although Paul struggles with fundamental concepts like adding two single-digit numbers, his mind is brilliant when it comes to understanding the concept of God, praying, and dying. Paul has always loved attending Immanuel Baptist Church and has been very dedicated in his attendance throughout his lifetime. And, up until February 2012, the same preacher pastored the small country church. Paul loves Pastor Bob Davies and his wife Diane; they have been pivotal in praying for his health over the last thirty years.

Paul has shared his love of music with his church congregation more than a few times with his rendition of his favorite old hymn, "I'll Fly Away." Paul loves music and he loves to share it with others. While the words remain unclear at times, he carries the tune in his head and his heart, making it very clear to others that he is singing to the Lord. Mom and Dad take Paul routinely to various nursing homes in our community to sing and visit with the residents. Paul compassionately walks from person to person, shaking hands and sharing his award-winning smile. If Mom isn't watching him too closely, Paul will drink the resident's coffee when left unattended on the table.

PRAYER

Besides glorifying God with music, Paul loves to pray, and he always prays in Jesus' name. When he was in his early twenties he would run up to the church podium immediately following the sermon to preach and pray to anyone remaining in the sanctuary. Oftentimes, I could only understand a few words, if any at all, because he would converse so rapidly. Although I could not understand most of what he preached, he had a twinkle in his eye and I am confident that God always understood every word Paul spoke.

Prayer is a significant part of Paul's life, and he will not begin a meal until the prayer has been said. I picked him up from work one time and he wanted me to sneak him a Happy Meal from McDonald's (without Mom's knowledge, of course). As I grabbed the food from the drive-up window, I excitedly handed him his Happy Meal. I explained that it was alright if he wanted to eat his meal in the car while we drove through the parent pick-up line to collect my three children from school. Paul quickly gave me a look of pure disappointment. He wanted to say a prayer, and he didn't want me to be distracted with driving. If he was going to pray, he wanted the prayer to be heartfelt and not simply a formality before consuming his food. The lesson I learned from him that day is to truly take time to thank God, and to do it with an undistracted heart.

Another aspect of prayer that I learned from Paul throughout his life is to pray with a pure heart and expectation that God will answer. He is also blessed with the gift of patience when it comes to praying. Growing up with a family of nine and a single income, money was often tight. Dad has only had a handful of trucks in the last forty years and most of them were older models with rust. Dad was a builder and wanted a truck that he could use without worry of scratching or denting. Paul, on the other hand, wanted Dad's truck to be brand new, perfectly clean, and Christmas red. For most of my life, Paul always prayed for Dad to get a new truck, even though Dad was happy with what he had. Paul continued to pray and wait patiently for almost forty years, and his prayers eventually came true.

When Dad retired from building homes, he also retired his old truck. Dad searched online for the perfect red truck that he knew Paul always wanted. Dad found one that matched Paul's description exactly and they purchased it. Watching Paul ride in the truck still draws me close to tears when I think about how God heard and answered his prayers. Paul had waited patiently and prayed without ceasing. He never got mad at God for not answering his prayers earlier. Paul proudly showed everyone Dad's new truck and called it Dad's Christmas truck because it was the perfect red. Once that prayer was answered he started praying for Mom to get a new Christmas car, but this time he didn't have to wait so long. Now all of their vehicles are red!

On special occasions Paul attended our fifth oldest brother, Tim's, church where he was pastoring. He would ask Paul to close his sermon in prayer. Watching Paul stand tall and proud, you could see clearly his direct connection to our Heavenly Father. When Paul prays, he prays purely from his heart, with little concern for who is hearing or what they might think. One humorous side to Paul's personality and prayer is that he will ask the shyest person at a gathering to pray aloud for everyone before the meal begins. He has an uncanny sense of who would be the most embarrassed in any situation. If you don't like to speak, let alone pray publically, hide at the next family gathering!

DYING

In 1978 we lost our Grandfather, and Paul began asking my parents questions about dying. He was only nine years old, but he understood that death meant leaving, and my parents explained to him that there was a place where Jesus lives called heaven. Paul assumed because Grandpa had white eyebrows and white hair when he died, that they were prerequisites for dying. He would ask my parents repeatedly when he could have white hair and eyebrows so he could go see Grandpa in Heaven.

Paul has danced a fine line between heaven and earth many times in his life, and he is excited for his turn to go to heaven. Paul is not afraid to die; in fact, he doesn't understand why he can't go to heaven right now. Often when he is very sick, he will point to his eyebrows and then point upwards, asking if his eyebrows are white yet. Dad always responds, "Not yet, Paul.", and Paul will start talking about all of his favorite animals that he hopes to see in heaven that have passed away some day.

He begins his list with Max, our beloved childhood Newfoundland puppy, who saved Paul from our busy road by pulling him by the pants and safely to the front porch of our home. Max also helped Paul get home when he wandered too far into the woods. Next he lists our German Shepherd Dog, Spot, who loved to fight any dog daring enough to walk past him. Then, he lists the people in his life that have passed away who he wants to see again, starting with Steve (brother number two), Grandmothers Ruth and Doris, and Grandfathers Ted and Woody. Although Grandpa Woody left this world in 1977, Paul has never forgotten him in heaven.

Our family was devastated when Steve passed away on February 17th, 2010 from pneumonia and complications of heart disease. Paul in particular had a bond with Steve that he has never experienced with anyone else—partly because Steve could "speak" Paul's language. It was amazing to listen to the two of them carry on a conversation. Steve had perfected the way Paul enunciated words and could communicate endlessly with Paul, while the rest of us conversed with him in short, simple sentences.

Paul talked about Steve going to heaven and sang "I'll Fly Away" at Steve's funeral in a passionate, gospel voice. Paul helped me deal with the loss of our brother, reminding me that Steve was in heaven with Max, Spot, and our grandparents. One time he told me that Steve was "all gone now" and smiled as he pointed upwards. On occasion, Paul will tell us that he sees Steve and points up in the air and sometimes waves. Who are we to say what he is able to see and understand? I think Paul understands a lot more about heaven and God than most people living on earth. I find this astounding because again, he is not able to understand simple math problems, but he comprehends the more complicated issue of death. When Paul stood on the stage at his best friend and brother's funeral, he wasn't crying. He was celebrating that Steve was no longer in pain and that he finally got to take his turn and go to heaven. Paul healed the hearts of so many people during the funeral service; at least twenty five people joined him on the stage with their voices and various musical instruments to celebrate Steve's life.

Paul was not angry with God for taking Steve, and while he misses him terribly, he understands that he doesn't need to say goodbye to Steve forever. However, just like anyone else, he has his moments with grief where he misses Steve unbearably and cannot stop crying or talking about him. Mom and Dad listen to him patiently and remind him that he will see Steve again. Once they start talking about heaven, he calms down. It is still very difficult for him to go to a hospital because he thinks of Steve and cannot stop asking Mom and Dad about heaven.

Regardless of others' beliefs about death and dying, Paul is constant in his belief that there is a heaven and that we as Christians will all meet up there together someday. He doesn't fear death, but embraces the idea that this world is temporary. Paul believes that family is important and that we should take every opportunity to say "I love you" and to hug and kiss our loved ones.

Paul doesn't just say goodbye when one of us leaves him, he hugs and kisses us until we see the twinkle in his eyes that shows us his pure, unconditional love. A person may have a lot of material wealth and intelligence on this earth, but what good does that do for him or her if he or she fails at showing love towards their friends, neighbors, family, or even strangers? If Paul left this world today, he would depart having already given hugs and kisses to each one of us the last time we were together. He doesn't ever miss the opportunity to show affection.

CHAPTER FIVE

Movies, Music, and More

"Sing to him a new song: play skillfully,
and shout for joy."
—Psalm 33:3

Paul has heavily influenced those around him with his passion for various music and movie artists. Paul's tastes are varied but, as with his church, he has been consistent and loyal to his favorites in movies and music throughout the years. My three children, along with all of Paul's other nieces and nephews, have grown to share this enthusiasm with him; thereby inspiring a new generation!

THE CHIPMUNKS

First and foremost, Paul loves Christmas music. Growing up, Christmas music bellowed out loudly from his bedroom year round. My only issue was that he frequently repeated the same song for hours each day. He loves music when he is happy, mad, angry, or sad, and he depends on it for a release of whatever emotions he carries throughout his day.

For example, one entire summer we had to listen to Alvin and the Chipmunks' Christmas album! As young as I was (a fourth grader) I remember thinking if I never heard that song again, it would still be too soon! Now that I no longer see through the eyes of a fourth grader, I actually smile when I hear the Chipmunks grace the radio waves during the Christmas season. I don't know exactly what it was about that album that Paul loved so much—maybe when Alvin gets yelled at by his music manager/guardian, Dave—but he listened his way through several copies of that tape.

TOM SAWYER

During my fourth grade year, Paul's obsession for music shifted to the vinyl record player and the constant scratching of the needle across the vinyl record drove me crazy! During this musical phase, he became obsessed with the 1973 version of *A Musical Adaptation of Mark Twain's Tom Sawyer*. His favorite was "The River Song." He repeatedly listened to the following verses, and could recite them from memory:

River runs warm in the summer sun,
River runs cold when the summer's done
But a boy's just a dreamer
By the riverside
'Cause the water's too fast
And the water's too wide . . .

. . . And a boy's gonna grow
To a man
To a man,
Only once in his life
Is he free
Only one golden time
In his life
Is he free

This song made me feel so sad for Tom Sawyer. I didn't like to hear it and couldn't understand why Paul enjoyed the song so much. But now, as an adult, I understand that like Tom Sawyer, Paul was turning from a boy into a man and I believe he understood a deeper meaning of the song as a fourteen-year-old boy. Recently, as my siblings and I were reminiscing about the good ole Tom Sawyer days—we remembered how Paul would mimic Tom's Aunt Polly scolding him to get ready for supper. Later, I picked Paul up from Comprehensive Services (his work site) because he was going to spend an hour or so hanging out with my family. After we picked the kids up from school and were driving home, I randomly started to sing the chorus of "The River Song." With perfect timing and pure shock to me, Paul remembered word for word Aunt Polly's lines.

With tears in my eyes and my children's laughter and amazement enveloping the car, we drove to my house, where Dad was working on my bathroom. Paul went upstairs to give Dad a hug and kiss, and I began to sing the song. Dad probably thought I lost my mind but I wanted to surprise him so that he could also experience how Paul remembered the timing and the words to the song so perfectly. To my embarrassment, Paul just stared at me after I finished the verse as if I had lost my mind!

Again, the children laughed uncontrollably and my son Braden said "Uncle Paul, Mom will give you $1.00 [his favorite denomination of money!] if you say your lines." This time as I sang the song, still feeling a little foolish, when Paul, on cue, perfectly recited the lines with a proud smile as long as the Mississippi River spreading over his face. Dad gave an emotional hug to Paul, who was simply proud of the fact that he made everyone laugh.

To collect stories and share memories with my family, I started a closed Facebook page called Being Bear: Things for My Book. It brought so much pleasure to all of us as we fondly recollected the memories that Paul brought us through his journey with Tom Sawyer. Tim (brother number 5) found "The River Song" on YouTube, so we played it for Paul. Watching him listen to the song again made his face shine with delight. Amazingly, he appeared to love the song as much as he did twenty-eight years ago.

BEACH BOYS

Another all-time, musical favorite of Paul's is the Beach Boys. As a child, I felt like I was growing up in California because of how much the Beach Boys sang about it and how much we listened to them. Paul expected a Beach Boys tape from Santa every Christmas—that was basically all that he wanted. Although he had multiple copies of the albums, rarely did a Christmas pass where he did not get some sort of new Beach Boys cassette tape. Dad laughed when he recalled seeing a large box of Paul's tapes in their barn that were worn and damaged; naturally they consisted mainly of the Beach Boys.

MUSICAL ADAPTATIONS

One humorous characteristic about Paul and music is how he can hear things in the song slightly different than what is actually sung. For example, our sister-in-law Cathy recalled when she first started dating my brother Mark (the third-oldest brother) how Paul would sing a Huckleberry Hound song that started out with the words, "Bark, bark, bark, Bark" but Paul would actually sing it "Mark, Mark, Mark, Mark." Paul would sing it to Mark teasingly many times over.

MARCHING BANDS

Paul also has a love for marching-band music. As a young boy, he loved the fact that our oldest brother Dave played the trumpet in the school marching band. During that time Dave would wear a tall hat equipped with chin strap and a purple and white feather sticking out of the top. Paul was saddened if a band played on TV or at a high-school event, and the band members did not wear his idea of an official headdress. His love for the marching band earned him his own trumpet, and eventually a tuba and a marching band hat with a plume (I found it at an antique store and it mysteriously disappeared . . . Mom?). The band was such an influential part of Paul's life that he coined the term "band haircut" for the type of hair cut that he wanted to wear. I assume it was because the marching band practiced out on the field in full sun for hours that most of the boys wore their hair closely cut, but Paul identified that as a significant attribute of being a real band member.

Paul gets very excited that two of my children play in the middle school band now and he reminds them often that he wants to attend another concert soon. One particular quality of Paul that I cherish is that in his mind, he is at the school concert watching superstars play together in a school band. He loves watching the children perform, just as much as he enjoys attending the Indianapolis Symphony Orchestra at Christmas time.

He usually puts things into perspective; often life moves so quickly that school band concerts can become just another event that I need to make sure we are all prepared for. Without words, Paul helps me to refocus on the important things in life, to take the time to enjoy the moment, and to forget about life's distractions.

THE AIR TRUMPET

One thing that none of us could ever fully understand was why Paul, when he would get upset, would pretend to play the trumpet while he hopped around in a circle. He would also yell the sound of his air trumpet, something like, "BU-NUH-NUH-NUH-NUH-NUH-NUH-NUH." At times when he was upset, music was the only catharsis for him. And judging by how much he would calm down after playing his air trumpet, I can say with confidence that this technique worked for him. He didn't get mad that often, but when he did, the air trumpet was played!

TELEVISION FAVORITES

During Paul's childhood, television shows were essential to him. We grew up watching *Batman*, *The Incredible Hulk*, *The Dukes of Hazzard*, *The Three Stooges*, *The A-Team*, and Chuck Norris's *Walker, Texas Ranger*. Being the only girl in a household of all male siblings, I rarely had too much say regarding TV shows. Thankfully one of my brothers loved *The Little House on the Prairie* as much as I did, so we claimed the TV for one hour each day.

MOVIES

In the mid-eighties the Tesmer clan advanced in the technological world by buying a VCR and Paul's love for movies bloomed. Like music, he would find one movie and then watch it until the tape wore so thin it would snap. I always felt sorry for Paul when this happened because the movies meant so much to him. Eventually Mom and Dad would replace the broken movie with another copy, but they at least gave us a small break from having it in the house.

THE "F" BOMB

My siblings and I recalled some of the movies we all promised never to watch again when we moved out on our own; we had seen or heard them so many times they were inscribed into our minds forever. *The Breakfast Club* quickly hit the top of the list. Paul loved this movie—one scene in particular. Because of this, the movie was quickly banned from our house.

His favorite part of the movie occurred in a high school library, where five detention students served time on a Saturday. The principal stopped in long enough to warn one of the students, "The next time I come in here I'm cracking skulls." As the principal slowly exits, the student yells "F—you." One day while the brothers were at home play wrestling, one of them said the infamous quote "The next time I come in here I'm cracking skulls." Perfectly on cue, clearly, and at full volume, Paul chimed the response.

The house was silent, the boys were stunned, and nobody moved until they could confirm that Mom didn't hear what came out of Paul's mouth. Unfortunately for them, she did. She quickly banned the movie from the house. Like typical teenage boys, and only if Mom was nowhere around, they would casually say the quote to see if they would get a response from Paul. My brothers and cousins would even prompt Paul with this quote in the men's bathroom at church of all places! I knew better than to test Paul's memory even twenty-five years later; I have full faith that he would recall the phrase flawlessly.

CHEVY CHASE

One actor that Paul adored was Chevy Chase and his *Vacation* movie series. The original *Vacation* has a few inappropriate scenes, so, Mom was wise and taped it from the TV where the language was cleaned up and the nudity removed. I had to watch various parts of that movie every morning of my entire high school career.

Paul's favorite scenes include Chevy Chase picnicking with his family while flirting with the ever-beautiful Christie Brinkley, and eating a sandwich that the dog had "marked." To this day, when Paul becomes hyper, usually if he sneaks a

Coke or coffee, he will cross his legs and bounce up and down while mimicking Chevy Chase eating a sandwich in that movie.

Another of his favorite parts also features Christie Brinkley (do you see the one main theme here?) flirtatiously asking Chevy (Clark Griswold) to jump into the pool and join her in skinny dipping, while his wife and children were upstairs in their motel room. Clark spreads his arms and claps his hands repeating the phrase, "This is crazy, this is crazy!" before jumping into the freezing cold pool. Again, on a day when Paul is feeling pretty good and there is water around, he will jump into the pool clapping his hands and repeating, "This is crazy, this is crazy!" followed by Paul's version of a loud scream. He is usually smiling too big, however, to produce a very loud scream. Perhaps certain interests, like pretty blond women, remain totally unaffected by Downs!

BEAR

I lovingly gave Paul the nickname "Bear" from the title of a movie. As much as Paul loves to watch and rent movies, he has never been able to drive himself to the local video store and rent whatever he wants. But one evening when I was in middle school, the telephone rang and the caller wanted to speak to Paul. I handed the phone to him. Out of curiosity I butted my ear up against the phone so that I could suss out the caller's needs. Paul answered, "Hello." The caller responded, "Hi Paul! Your reservation for the movie *Bear* is in and you can pick it up whenever you like." Paul hung up the phone with a self-important smile, proud of having received a call. I laughed because I knew that he didn't reserve a movie, but Video Heaven called him a few more times that day notifying him that his movie was in.

With an excess of time and curiosity on our hands, we rented the movie to find out how it had been reserved under his name. It turned out not to be very good. Paul was disappointed, too. That is the moment that I said to him, "It's okay, Bear, you can rent another one sometime." He immediately told Mom that I called him Bear, and that playfully fueled my desire to tease him more. After awhile, he didn't seem to mind the nickname, and I had grown accustomed to calling him Bear. We never did figure out who reserved the movie using his name and telephone number at Video Heaven, but he is still lovingly called Bear today.

INFECTIOUS INTERESTS

Paul's passion for music and movies is so contagious that he has shared this love with many others. My children have watched every episode of *Walker, Texas Ranger* and have seen all of the original episodes of *The Incredible Hulk* that I watched with Paul as a child. Paul's influence was apparent when my two boys bought Chuck Norris t-shirts, not because Mr. Norris was cool in their teenage world, but because they associate wonderful memories of watching the episodes with their uncle. Simply put, Paul's passions are infectious to those of us around him.

Paul was not expected to live but a few days after he was born on May 28, 1969. God clearly had different plans! Our family will be forever grateful to Riley Children's Hospital, and to Dr. Fred Haggerty, Paul's family doctor, for working diligently to save his life many times.

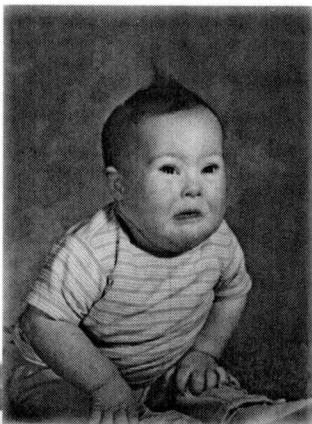

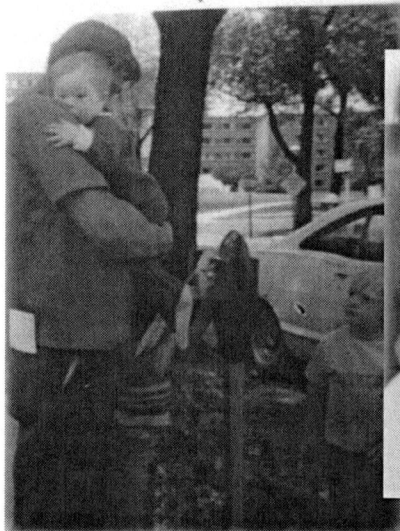

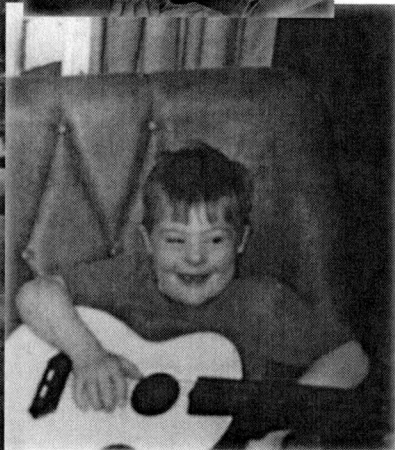

Another trip to Riley Children's Hospital. Pneumonia has been a huge problem for Paul since birth. Mom and Dad had the three older children, Dave, Steve, and Mark in tow on this visit.

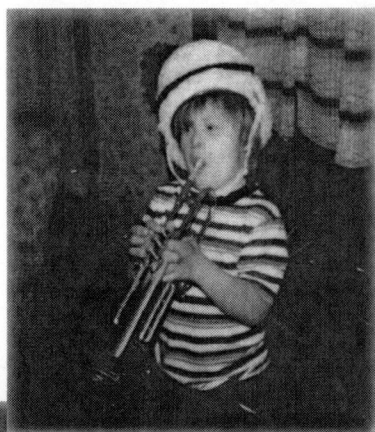

Dave, our oldest brother, was in the Greencastle Marching Band in High School. Paul would wear Dave's hat and march around the house playing the trumpet.

Mark, Steve, Dave (back row) Joy, Matt, Tim, Paul (first row). Chirstmas Eve pajamas!

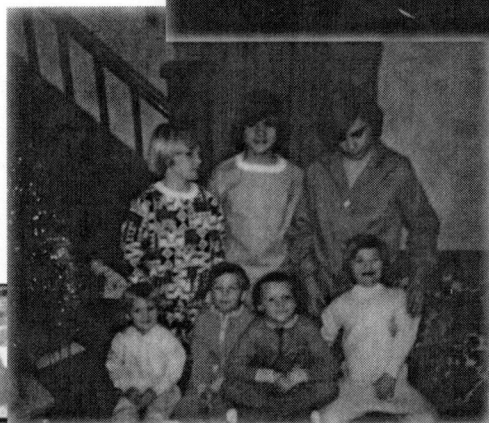

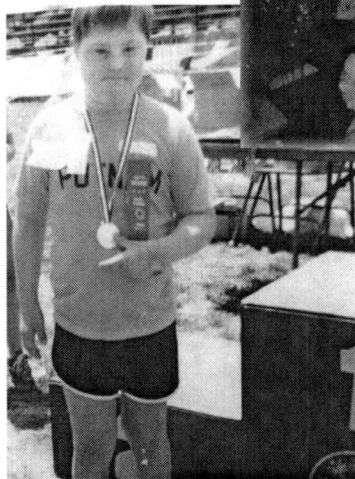

The Special Olympics has been a significant part of Paul's life.

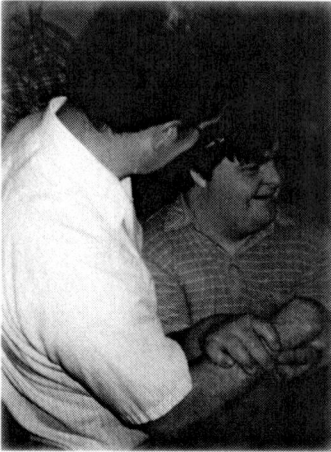

Paul being baptized by Pastor Bob Davies.

Paul loved his Newfoundland dogs, Max (black dog on the right) and Lady (black and white dog on the left). The mailman witnessed Max pull Paul out of middle of a busy intersection in Florida, and recounted the amazing story to my parents. Max was especially aware of what Paul was allowed to do and what he wasn't allowed to do.

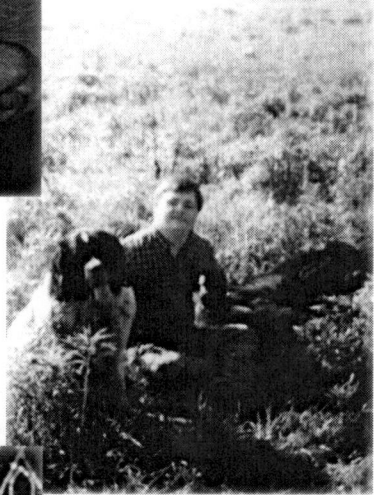

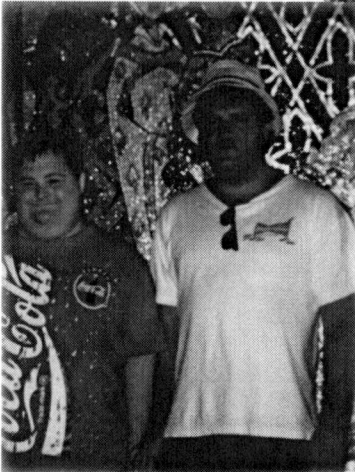

Steve, our second oldest brother, was Paul's best friend. Steve could "talk" like Paul and Paul loved communicating with Steve in their own language. Steve passed away in 2010, and Paul continues to remind us daily that Steve is with Jesus in Heaven, with our Grandparents, and Spot, Max and Lady (his dogs).

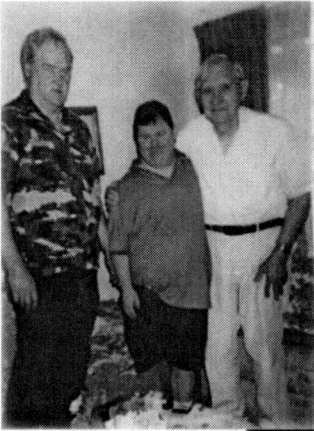

Paul loved Grandpa Ted. He loved to fly to Arizona to visit Grandpa and he expected Dad and Mom to rent a red rental car every time. After Grandpa passed away, Paul reminded us that Grandpa is in Heaven!

When our brother Steve ran for judge, Paul couldn't wait to be in the parade. Our entire family walked the parade route passing out candy and fliers, while Paul sat in the back of the truck dressed as Uncle Sam!

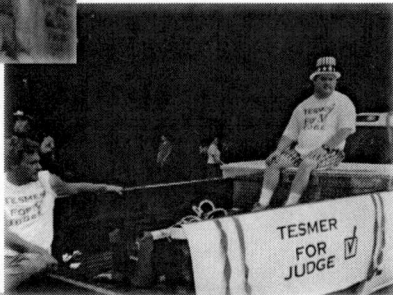

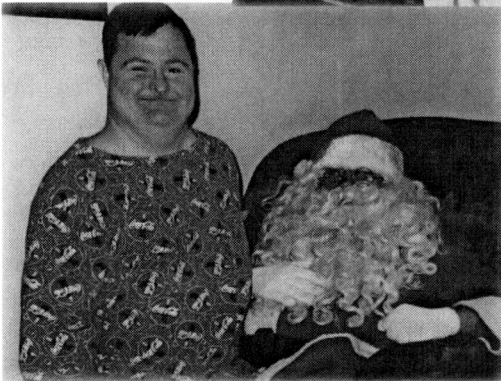

In Paul's view, one is never too old to sit on Santa's lap! Santa visits Paul at home each Christmas where he delivers a few presents before the 25th! Each year Paul wants to see the Reindeer . . . I have yet to figure that one out!

Paul loves his nieces and nephews. He is especially excited that he is going to be a great-uncle next year! He loves to hold the children on his lap and tell them about the corn and the beans. Emeline is like a daughter to him. Arianna, in the background, is constantly entertained by Paul's wonderful sense of humor.

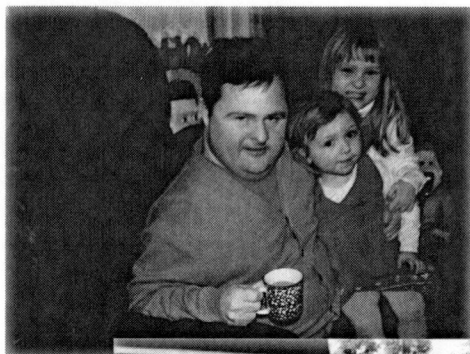

We have a huge family! This picture was taken at Paul's 40th birthday party. We decorated Christmas trees, displayed Christmas decorations, and even Santa came to celebrate!

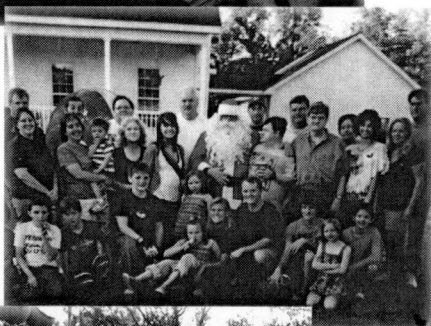

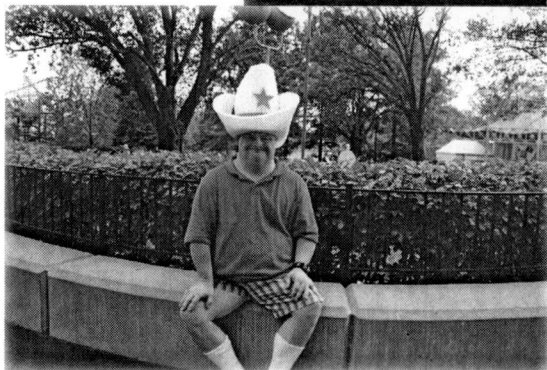

Paul got such a kick out of this hat. Our entire family went to King's Island, a theme park, and our nephew Jerry won this hat. Paul loved it so much that he wanted his picture taken with the hat. He didn't want to wear it for very long because he was very worried about his hair getting messed up. He loves his hair to be short. and always combed.

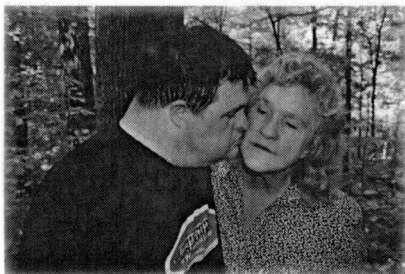

Mom has devoted her entire life to Paul's healthcare. Paul would not be alive today if it were not for her. We joke that she should have a medical license because she has had to learn more about the human body than a doctor attending medical school. Paul doesn't like to be away from Mom and Dad for more than a few hours. I think he understands that they have both been his lifeline.

Paul is truly one of my best friends in life. My love and admiration for him is beyond words. Paul can ride a two-wheeled bike, but this one has a basket so he can carry his water bottles in it. This is the bike that Paul and I wrecked when I was on the bike with him. As he soared over my head, I twisted upward to grab ahold of him in an attempt to protect him from the concrete ravine. I am proud to say that he landed on me and didn't get hurt. I on the otherhand, suffered a crack in my kneecap and injured my wrist, and shoulder. As I held onto Paul on the side of the road, him dangling a few feet over large rocks, our amazing neighbor ran to our rescue! Paul won't even let me touch his bike anymore in fear that I will wreck it again. His wisdom is spot-on!

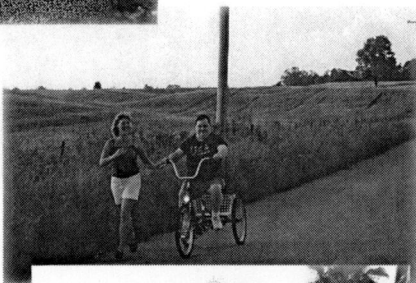

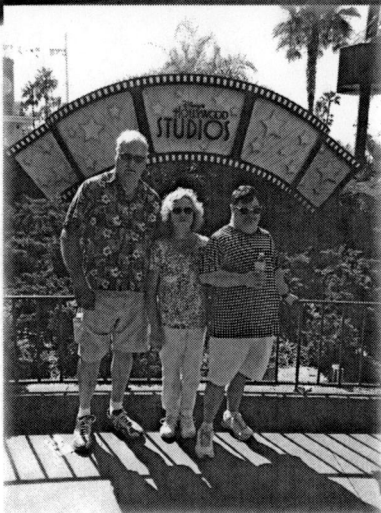

The heros of my life. Dad, Mom, and Paul at Disney World's Hollywood Studios in June, 2012.

CHAPTER SIX

Work Ethic

*"The harvest is plentiful but the workers
are few."*
—Matthew 9:38

Work is a high priority in Paul's life, next to church and family. His work ethic is so strong that he could write a self-help book for people wanting to develop one. I have observed that he lives by the following work rules.

Paul's Ten Work Rules

1. Show up to work on time and with a smile.
2. Unless you are dying (literally), don't miss work.
3. Don't waste money eating out every day; have your mom pack your lunch and your drinks for the day.
4. Save your money and don't make excuses.
5. Take pride in what you do and clean up after yourself.
6. Do everything to the best of your *ability* without complaining.
7. Be nice to your coworkers; they are your second family.
8. Even if you have a boss that does not respect you, show and teach him or her unconditional love.
9. Accept every job request with a "yep."
10. If a coworker leaves a drink on the table, help him or her out and drink it!

The Trash Man

As a young boy Paul dreamed of becoming a trash man. In the late seventies, our house on Howard Street would be moderately calm and then erupt with enthusiastic shouts of excitement, followed by the sound of feet running hastily to the window. We all knew this meant that the trash truck was on our street and would soon stop in front of our house to empty our trash cans.

To Paul, the sanitation workers were equivalent to rock stars. He would press his face against the living room window and continue shouting and waving until the truck moved slowly down the road. With Paul's penchant for tidiness, he also relished the days that Dad would clean out the basement garage and let us ride along in the truck to our local refuse handling station.

Paul's influence becomes again evident. How many five-year-old girls looked forward to piling into a truck filled with a bed of trash and a bunch of boys for a journey to the dump? And yet, I remember precisely the rush I felt in my belly when Dad announced it was time to load up in his old green truck. The excitement was intense as Paul proudly took his spot in the front seat next to Dad, anticipating his venture to evacuate the trash.

He so loved picking up trash that somebody gave him an old grocery cart to push around our yard and fill with litter from the ground. He would sport a ball cap and gloves and clean up the earth, one piece of refuse at a time. He loved his grocery cart and was obviously proud of his trash collection and clean working environment.

Signature "P"

Paul learned to write the letter "P" for his signature when he was in elementary school. I remember Mom always kept a pad of paper next to the phone to take messages that came in for Dad during the day for his construction company. It was always comical and somewhat wearisome to grab the notebook of paper to promptly jot down a prospective customer's information and discover that once again every page in the pad was filled with P's. He is very proud of his signature. He used to grace my homework pages with his official autograph if I carelessly left my binder out on the table!

Comprehensive Services

Paul started working at Comprehensive Services when he was five years old. Chuck Schroedar started building the program from a preexisting base and worked diligently to fund and develop the program for special needs clients. Comprehensive Services now has a financial agreement with some local factories to outsource such things as packing screws and washers into bags for them. Jobs like this give the clients specific work to look forward to and in which their success is attainable.

Paul's coworkers are like a second family to him. Throughout the years, he has worked alongside his buddies and they help watch over him. One friend in particular that Paul has known since he was a child is Robyn. Robyn is like a mother to Paul when he is at work. They met each other in elementary school, and Robyn clearly loved Paul from the beginning. Each morning when he walks into the workshop at Comprehensive Services, Robyn rushes over to him with a smile on her face and offers to help him put his lunchbox and thermos into the refrigerator. She is the only coworker that he will dance with at the annual Valentine's Day dance.

Mom and Dad have met some of the nicest and most selfless people working for Comprehensive Services that watch over the clients. Unfortunately the pay in the social services industry is minimal and the turnover rate can be quite high. This industry is not for the faint of heart, since some of the client's' needs can require heavy lifting and special care.

Our family will forever be grateful to Comprehensive Services staff for their great efforts that they have demonstrated throughout the years of Paul's attendance. Teddy, Paul's surrogate grandmother at work, treats Paul with loving care that only the best of grandmothers can provide. And Judy, whose unrelenting efforts ensure that all clients who want to participate in Special Olympics have the opportunity. Jaimie and Betty, two of Paul's personal staff favorites, take Paul bowling, on picnics, and out to eat, socializing with him as his surrogate sisters. Finally, Barb, Marilyn, Donna, and Chuck, who work with my parents frequently to continue to maintain a superior program for all clients.

SIMPLY MISBEHAVING

As much as Paul enjoys work and takes pride in his success, there have also been occasions where he has made it difficult for the staff members to keep him safe. Mom recalls the time that she went to pick Paul up from work just to find out that he snuck out the back door and climbed fifteen feet up a satellite tower behind the work building.

Another difficult time for the staff occurred when Paul wanted to go outside and they did not have enough people to supervise all of the clients; so he was told no. Paul's stubbornness kicked in, and he watched carefully for an opportunity to sneak out. As a master escape artist, it didn't take long before he approached the house next door to the center. After breaking a window out of the house, the staff found him trying to get inside so he could watch television. Needless to say, Dad stopped by after his long day at work and repaired the damages to the window.

Paul has an excellent memory and if he watches something done once, or if he visits a place, he seems to never forget it. One day while at work he crossed Greencastle's busiest highway to visit my sister-in-law at a local insurance company. She recalls looking up and seeing Paul smugly standing in the doorway telling her, "Hi." Thankfully she was able to drive him back to work to a much-concerned staff.

The last issue Paul has yet to overcome at work is his bad habit of drinking people's drinks that they leave unattended. Paul has severe acid reflux and is therefore only allowed milk, tea, and water. On rare occasions, Mom will allow him to have a small Coke or Sprite to curb a craving, but it usually ends up hurting his chest afterward. Many clients and staff members set their coffee or soda cups down only to pick them up and find the cup empty.

It is no longer a secret who the phantom drink stealer is at work, so most workers and clients try to more closely manage their beverages. However Paul outsmarted them one day when one of the staff members prepared a meal supplement for a young lady in a service chair with a feeding tube. The staff member carefully prepared the supplement and momentarily set it down to prepare the feeding tube. When she went to grab the supplement it had been emptied. Paul was the suspect, and his milk mustache convicted him as the drink thief!

Paul continues to this day to try to walk off and discover interesting things. He is usually pretty good about asking for permission first, but if he doesn't like the answer he is given, he usually tries to do it anyway. The center has worked diligently with Mom to make sure that Paul has scheduled daily activities when he is not working in the workshop to satisfy his wanderlust.

Paul requires clean spaces and energy conservation in any space that he occupies. If a floor looks dirty, he finds a broom and cleans it up. He keeps his bedroom and music room spotless, and he loves to vacuum the house.

Do It Right the First Time

I appreciate when he comes over to my house and wants to vacuum the floor because he spends about an hour taking his time to clean one area at a time. He doesn't leave a speck of dirt anywhere. He also loves to use the steam mop on my kitchen floor. It seems like every board on the floor gets a thirty swipe turn before he moves on to the next one. If he is going to do something, he wants it done right!

Paul's second Work Rule, "Unless you are dying, don't miss work" is no joke. Paul has demanded that he make money at work while dealing with reoccurring illnesses like sinus infections, pneumonia, and eye ulcers. He doesn't always win the battle for work if Mom thinks it isn't a good idea, but he always gives it his best shot. Paul is persistent and stubborn, and if he has it in his mind that he is going to work, he will try Mom's endless patience until, eventually, one of them gives in.

Paul works without excuses or complaints, which is often more than I can say for myself. It amazes me how he has mastered a highly dedicated work ethic, while many Americans without diagnosable disabilities have not. We can all gain knowledge from his great and humble wisdom.

CHAPTER SEVEN

Flying High

"They will soar on wings like eagles; they will run and not grow weary, they will walk and not be faint."
—Isaiah 40:31

Paul looks forward to family vacation every year. Vacation, as defined by Paul, consists of full sun, an ocean, and a hotel with a full service breakfast. Paul loves flying in airplanes and has always loved to spot planes in the sky. When he sees a plane above, he assumes it is vacation-bound.

AIRPLANES AND COKE

I have had the privilege of flying with Paul a few times; he makes modest, almost unseen aspects of the experience seem utterly magical through his pure appreciation for and anticipation of them. For instance, a few months before any vacation, he begins anticipating the flight attendant handing him a Sprite so he can drink it on the plane. He becomes so eager for the event that he will stop strangers in the grocery store to tell them that soon he will get to drink a "Coke" on the plane. Paul refers to all soft drinks as "Coke"; this must surely be related to Coke's marketing of Santa Claus during the Christmas season.

Another anticipatory action Paul takes months prior to his trip, is to spread his arms straight out on each side of his body and then begin waving them like the wings of an airplane. He will approach the person nearest him in whatever location (church, grocery store, movie theatre, etc.) and perform his wing rotation. He does this in part because of the thrill leading up to the trip, and partly, I believe, to reaffirm that he is going on an airplane soon. The remarkable thing about his love for planes is that our grandfather held his pilot's license and managed a small airport when our father was growing up. Paul never saw Grandpa Ted in this capacity, so I can only assume his love for aviation is genetic.

THE BIG TAKE-OFF

Once on the airplane, the excitement that Paul exudes takes an ordinary flight and makes it extraordinary. As the flight attendant reviews the information cards, Paul watches attentively—eyes squinted, thumb touching his lip, and his index finger pushing the skin around the corner of his eye upward. This is what I call his philosopher's pose. It surfaces when he experiences stress, sickness, excitement, or any heightened emotion.

As the plane begins to accelerate, Paul reminds "Mommy and Daddy" (that is what he calls our parents unless he is in a funny mood and refers to them as Jerr and Marcia) that they are about to take off. At the point where the plane is in an upward incline, about to leave the ground and ascend into the sky, he can no longer contain his excitement; on cue every single time he yells "YEEE-HAAAAW." Once the plane lands, Paul faithfully claps for the captain of the plane in celebration of a job well done. Paul is and will always be very consistent when it comes to his aviation, transportation routine.

No Vacation from Illness

No matter where Paul goes on vacation, Mom and Dad have to observe him vigilantly at all times regarding his health and immune system. Although vacations are exciting and relaxing for Paul, Mom and Dad have frequented various hospitals on their journeys with him over the years. Consequently, they like to plan trips with a maximum of six days so they are not trapped in another state, far away from his regular doctors for very long.

Once when Mom and Dad took Paul to Mesa, Arizona to visit our grandfather, Ted, Paul became seriously ill in a matter of hours. Being in a cramped hotel room and without the amenities of home was quite wearisome. When Dad called me to help him rearrange their flights, I realized for the first time how terrifying it actually was to travel with Paul and the infinite responsibilities they take on when he becomes sick.

One major issue that presented itself immediately was that the airlines could not find seats on any flights departing for Indiana. To top it off, the hospital refused to care for Paul because his insurance from Medicaid and Medicare would not accept payment responsibilities out of his state of residency. When they finally boarded the plane to fly home three days later, Paul's comfortable transport became paramount. He was having considerable issues with vomiting and diarrhea. Dad and Mom held the small air sickness bag for Paul, while he lost dangerous amounts of fluids from his body.

Paul cannot be left alone when he is weak and sick, so Dad crammed himself into the airplane bathroom with Paul each time they were fortunate enough to make it there in time. Airplane lavatories are not built for a man like our six-foot-four-inches tall father to comfortably fit into, let alone when you add another 190-pound body in there. I get claustrophobic just imagining it. Add to the recipe the unfortunate odor of sickness that was emitted into the enclosed space over 32,000 feet in the air!

A WINDOW SEAT

On vacations Mom and Dad try to let Paul feel as relaxed as possible without hovering over him like a helicopter. They will show him highlights of the area they are visiting and ask him activities he would like to do or what he would like to explore further. I admire the way they value Paul's individual opinions and interests. They do have their limits, however, because Paul has very expensive taste and they are always on a tight budget!

Paul loves to take long car drives and watch the world go by from the glass of his air-conditioned car. Food is always a priority and he looks forward to the restaurants during vacation as much or more than the activities of the day. When Mom and Dad look for places of interest, they examine the necessities for our family, such as easily accessible bathrooms and shaded areas to take a break.

THE OCEAN'S EDGE

If water is near, Paul is, too! He loves the ocean and he loves sitting on the edge of the water, feeling the waves break against his legs and the sand pull against his body. Mom and Dad watch him closely, but accommodate his need for quiet time. He could sit there for hours if someone brought him food and drinks, but usually his hunger alerts him to retreat inside for lunch. He does not like to be hot, and his skin is fair, so Mom guides him back inside before he gets sun burned.

COCOA BEACH, FLORIDA

I warmly remember our trip in September 1996 when Mom, Dad, Paul, Brian, our ten-month-old son Brandon, my brothers, Steve (number two) and Tim (number five), along with my sister-in-law Kim, and I, flew to Cocoa Beach, Florida for a week to share a beach house. The beach house was small but had an enormous and beautiful glass window overlooking the Atlantic Ocean. We loved spending an entire week waking up to the beautiful view and Paul treasured Steve being there with him as the only bachelors on the trip!

That particular trip was amazing because Steve, who suffered from claustrophobia and agoraphobia, actually boarded the plane and left his contented surroundings to spend time with Paul. It was one of the most unselfish acts of his lifetime. Paul loved it that Mom and Dad took him and Steve to NASA's Kennedy Space Center and other fun places while the rest of us played on Cocoa Beach.

One day, the sun beat down with such intensity that Paul couldn't spend much time outside. So, Mom, Dad, and Steve took Paul on a drive down the coastline so he could enjoy the water while staying out of the acute heat. As they came to each beach beginning with the first, they would disembark from the car and walk up to the beach and take a look around. Things went smoothly until they got to the tenth beach. As they walked up the steps to check out the beach they noticed that many people were walking around naked. Although the beach sign clearly stated that bathing suits must be worn, it was obviously a locally accepted secret. Needless to say, they left quickly and decided they had seen enough beaches for the day.

HOLIDAY WORLD

One weekend trip several years later, our entire family went to an amusement park about three hours from home in Santa Claus, Indiana, called Holiday World. Paul loved Holiday World the moment he saw the massive Santa Claus statue towering at the front entrance. He attended a story time with Santa, but was disgruntled because Santa wasn't fully dressed in his winter red suit. The temperature was around ninety-five degrees that day, so we decided to take Paul to the water park to cool off. As Paul was going down one of the water slides, he didn't expect it to shoot him down into the water and wasn't prepared for the jolt. Even though I was waiting for him just inches away, he came so fast I couldn't help him. He came down hard and slammed his knee into the bottom of the pool with a force great enough to crack his knee cap. While his knee started swelling, he was dismayed that we might have to go home!

MAGICAL MEMORIES

Paul loves the food, fun, and experiences of vacations, but it doesn't take long before he begins to miss his home and his dogs. I get so much more out of vacations when we all go together, because Paul doesn't let small things go unnoticed. A drink on an airplane, shaking hands with strangers, watching the dolphins—it all seems more magical with him because he appreciates those things so much. As we now prepare for another trip to Disney World, Paul pulls out his new suitcase and rolls it around the house, fascinated that the wheels turn so easily. Even I feel excited now about how cool his suitcase rolls! Everything is simply magical!

CHAPTER EIGHT

Cleanliness Is Next to Godliness

*"Do you know that your body is a temple
of the Holy Spirit, who is in you, whom
you have received from God? You are not
your own; you were bought at a price.
Therefore honor God with our body."*
—*1 Corinthians 6:19*

Most people do not likely know that Paul is a clean
freak! If you leave your cup on the table for even a
second, Paul will both drink it and thoughtfully take
it to the kitchen. He cannot stand things being left
out of place. He also cannot stand lights left on in

an unoccupied room. Imagine the electricity savings in our world if everyone conserved as much energy as Paul!

ENERGY CONSERVATOR

Paul jokingly enjoys shutting the lights off on people in bathrooms in the name of energy conservation. He kept getting in trouble at work because he would notice that the women's bathroom light was on and he kept shutting it off. Of course he knows not to go in there, but he doesn't understand that the bathroom does not have any exterior windows and therefore puts any restroom users in total darkness!

DICK'S BARBER SHOP

Paul's first haircut came from Dick Asbell and their business relationship continues today. Paul is loyal! He does not like anyone cutting his hair besides Dick. As with everything else, Paul doesn't like the routine to change when he goes into the barber shop for his monthly cut. He waits patiently for Dick's barber chair to become vacant, and then he rushes into the seat. He always shakes Dick's hand, and lets Dick know that he is there to get a haircut. Afterwards, Dick gives Paul a few pieces of wrapped bubble gum and Dad pays for the haircut.

Paul does not like to let his hair grow out very much, and Mom and Dad will not hear the end of it until they take him back in for another haircut.

Because Paul demands that every dark brown hair on his head be in its rightful place, he becomes an easy target to be teased. Dave (brother number one) seems to get the most enjoyment out of sneaking up behind Paul and messing up his hair. Paul does this to me teasingly all of the time, but he does not like for it to be done to him! He quickly grabs a comb and, with perfect accuracy, combs his locks back into place.

Public Bathroom Routine

Paul is very particular about washing his hands. He refuses to pass a sink and miss an opportunity to stay clean. As he has gotten older, he has developed a few more steps to his bathroom routine that make the process a much longer one for sure!

Once my husband, then boyfriend, Brian, volunteered to take Paul into a public bathroom. Paul approached the urinals and proceeded to take care of business as Brian did the same. Brian was in a temporary position of not being able to move as he noticed Paul standing at the urinal beside him, tap the guy standing next to him on the shoulder to shake his hand. Brian tried explaining to Paul that it wasn't a good place to shake hands, but twenty years later, Paul still walks into a bathroom and sometimes grabs the person's shoulders while they are standing in front of the urinal and invites them to shake his hand. As Brian lovingly puts it, Paul doesn't really give "bystanders" at the urinal much of a choice but to shake his hand. He just wants to be friendly and greet people. He does not seem to understand the personal boundaries that public bathrooms have.

Once Paul greets his fellow rest room users and finishes his business at the urinal, he will not button or zip his pants until he is satisfied with his underwear placement. He will pull them all the way down and back up until he decides that they fit just right. Hurrying him along is futile because he has no problem with pulling his pants down anywhere to fix them! It is most efficient just to let him get them right where he wants them.

Once he is satisfied with his clothes he moves to the sink and will continue to greet those around him. He uses soap, scrubs his hands and lower arms, checks his hair, and washes his face. He prefers using electric hand dryers versus paper towels because he likes to dry his face as well. Finally, before leaving the bathroom, he does a final check in the mirror to make sure that not one hair is out of place.

THE NAKED GUN

One evening when we were younger and living at home, some of the boys were watching Leslie Nielsen's movie, *The Naked Gun*. In one scene, Lieutenant Frank Drebin (played by Mr. Nielsen) was speaking publicly with a microphone and proceeded to enter the bathroom with the microphone still activated. In the scene, Drebin sings in the stall while he uses the bathroom. Paul laughed at this scene and no one was surprised the next Sunday evening at church when Paul excused himself to the bathroom during the evening service. The rest of the congregation heard Paul singing from the men's bathroom. Dad was the first back there to see what was going on, just to find Paul reenacting Nielsen's scene perfectly, down to making circles in the toilet water with his stream! And, for good measure, he knocked on the bathroom door to announce he was coming back out to the sanctuary. This was the late 80's when he saw this movie and he has not forgotten about it today!

WATCH AND BILLFOLD

Paul refuses to leave the house unless he is wearing his wristwatch and his billfold is in his pocket. It does not matter if there is an emergency or if he is just running cookies into to town with Mom for the grandkids—the watch and billfold must be in place!

I enjoy when he comes over to my house because he has his own special routine there, too.

When Paul steps into my home, he immediately takes off his shoes. I have told him constantly that it is okay if he wants to leave them on, but he will not wear shoes in a house. Next, he walks into the living room and places his billfold and watch on a side table before making himself comfortable. Mom will try to tell him that they are only staying for a few minutes, but his routine behavior prevents him from deviating from his norm.

SPOTS ON!

Paul is an incredibly hard worker, even when the job entails getting dirty. However, if he is eating lunch and food or drink falls on his shirt, he will remove the shirt and get another one. Paul cannot stand to be untidy and spots on his shirts unnerve him. He is the same way with his white tennis shoes, too. He wants them to stay perfectly white and when he can no longer clean off the dirt spots, he will unrelentingly remind Mom that he needs new shoes. Once she thought that she would try black shoes to introduce a bit a variety. When the shoes came in the mail, he took one look at them and then one look at her before shaking his head emphatically, "No!" The next morning when he was dressing for work she noticed that he was putting on his old white tennis shoes instead of his new black ones. She reminded him that she bought him new shoes and when she went to look for them she couldn't find them anywhere.

After repeated questioning, Paul finally confessed the hiding spot as he brought the shoes to Mom. When they came to visit at my house, he pointed to his shoes and motioned his hand sign for "gone" or "away." I asked mom what he was saying because I knew how much he loved getting new shoes and she told me that he kept hiding the new black ones. A few days later Mom was again questioning Paul about where he hid the new shoes, and all he would say is, "All gone now!" Mom never found the black New Balance shoes and the suspicion is they went into the trash when she wasn't looking.

CLEAN SHAVEN

Paul is a man without a beard by choice. He cannot stand to have a five o'clock shadow, so Mom usually has to shave him at least once a day. Mom has learned that if Paul tells her that he wants shaved, she had better clear her schedule quickly or he will do it himself, which inevitably leads to razor burn, nicks, and blood. I remember in high school once when Paul wanted to be shaved while Mom was preparing for dinner. I volunteered to shave him for her, and I was amazed at how detailed the entire process actually was. Paul will not deviate from any routine; he likes to be shaved exactly like Mom shaves him or he will cry. I could not believe the trust in his eyes as I lathered his face with Gillette shaving cream and shaved away his five o'clock shadow.

Because of the pride Paul takes in his appearance, he will still dress nicely in his clean jeans or shorts and a clean t-shirt even if he is not leaving the house for the day. He will still comb his hair no fewer than fifteen times during that day, and he will continue to look in the mirror throughout the day to make sure he is keeping a presentable appearance. Not only that, but the house will remain tidy too!

CHAPTER NINE

The Naked Truth

*"These are the things that you do: Speak
the truth to each other, and render true
and sound judgment in your courts."*
—*Zechariah 8:16*

Honest Allusions

The following poem is written by me from Paul's perspective. These couplets illustrate the ideals by which he lives and, I think, are instructive for all of mankind.

I don't judge people by what they wear,
To be so judgmental doesn't seem fair!

I don't notice how much money you make,
I am honest and loving; I don't want to be fake!

If you are orange-skinned or even pale blue,
I want you to know, I'm just fine with you.

People lose sight of the moment right now,
And miss opportunities to help others out.

Stop making excuses, complaining, and crying,
Live a purposeful life, with no regrets or lying.

Turn up your music; hug your family and friends,
Because our time here is short and will certainly
end!

Ask yourself if you like being you and what you
should change,
Then take time to discover what you must
rearrange!

But if its money you are after, or a prestigious title
or two
All I can say, is it must *stink* being you!

MODESTY?

Paul is not modest by any means. This is, conceivably, due to the time spent in hospitals over the last forty-two years. Another possibility is that he is simply not ashamed, embarrassed, or self-conscious about his body. In fact, he is very proud of his round belly.

One of my all-time favorite memories with Paul occurred, again, at Holiday World, and, again, with Brian. Brian and I took Paul and our three children to the water park while Mom and Dad rested awhile in the shade. Arianna and I went into the ladies room to change into our bathing suits and Brian took our two boys and Paul into the men's room. After enjoying the water slides for a couple of hours, we were all exhausted and ready to return to dry clothes. Unfortunately, everyone else at the water park thought it was a fine idea to change at that time too, leaving the changing lines backed-up. To make things worse, bodies were packed shoulder to shoulder inside the small changing area.

While Brian was looking around the locker room for an open space where the guys could change their clothes, he noticed a group of men moving to one side or the other, dividing the room, like Moses parting the Dead Sea. When he looked around to see what was going on, he realized that Paul had taken off his swimming trunks and walked comfortably around the locker room totally naked, reaching out and shaking hands with strangers along the way. Brian and the boys saw an opportunity in the newly opened space and quickly followed behind Paul to change out of their soaked clothes!

When Arianna and I finally met the boys outside, Paul was noticeably proud that he had helped the boys promptly change clothes. And, the boys were tickled because they could not believe how fearless and courageously bold their uncle was to saunter so carefree and untroubled through a sea of people . . . completely undressed.

SECRETS REVEALED

There are so many things that I love about Paul, but most of all, I love that he is so honest and tells the truth! When our second brother Steve, started smoking in law school, he quickly became addicted to cigarettes. When Steve came home during a short break, Paul found him hiding outside the house smoking. It didn't take long for the truth to come out. In fact, at dinner that night Paul said, "Daddy, Steve smoke." He used hand gestures to ensure that his communication would be understood accurately.

JUST FLUSH IT

Another funny memory, which was not amusing to Mom and Dad at the time, was when Paul went through a phase of flushing random objects down the toilet. If something in the house showed up missing, Mom and Dad knew to ask Paul if he had flushed it down the toilet. He never lied; in fact, he would usually answer, "Yep!" One of the weirdest things he flushed was the TV remote, which made him frustrated at Mom because he couldn't change the channels without getting up from his chair anymore. During the flushing phase, he watched more full rolls of toilet paper go down the commode than my parents could afford!

HONESTY

Paul does not have a problem saying "No!" I have asked him many times if he would like to come over and watch a movie with us, and he will sometimes stubbornly shake his head and say "No." He loves hanging out with Mom and Dad, especially at night when he wants to be in his pajama pants and watching movies.

His complete honesty reminds me of the verse in the Bible where it says "Let your yes be yes and your no be no . . . James 5:12." It is hard to get too annoyed at someone who frankly tells you that they are guilty of flushing your favorite pen down the toilet! If only the rest of the world could be as honest!

CHAPTER TEN

What the World Can Learn

*Jesus replied, "Do not murder, do not
commit adultery, do not steal, do not
give false testimony, honor your father
and mother, and love your neighbor as
yourself."*
—*Matthew 19:18*

When I read this Bible verse I am convinced
of how much of the big picture Paul understands.
By actively living the commands of not murdering,
committing adultery, stealing, lying, honoring
parents, and loving neighbors, Paul models the

actions of a true Christian man. When I discussed with my family the possibility of documenting his life, we came up with the following life lessons by which Paul lives that might encourage others to live a happier, more wholesome life. "Love the Lord your God with all your heart and with all you soul and with all your mind. This is the first and greatest commandment . . ." Matthew 22:37

STAY AWAY FROM GODLESS CHATTER

One blessing that I believe Paul has in his life, as a result of his disability, is avoiding gossip. Consider the words that have exited mouths that have been used to hurt, deceive, or cut someone down. Paul has maintained integrity with his words and actions, without "godless chatter." 2 Timothy 2:16 reads, "Avoid godless chatter, because those who indulge in it will become more and more ungodly." This task would be difficult for most of us on an hourly basis, let alone over the course of a lifetime!

BE HAPPY WITH WHAT YOU HAVE

Paul loves money, but not in a worldly way. He takes pride in having earned as many one-dollar bills as he can pack into his billfold. He enjoys cashing his paycheck at the bank and having it remitted back in crisp, dollar bills. In fact, if given the choice of a one-hundred-dollar bill or a one dollar bill, he will most always choose the one-dollar bill.

He doesn't understand the value of different denominations of cash, but he does understand that money is necessary to purchase things. However, money does not rule his life or distract him from more important matters. Matthew 6:24 reminds us that ". . . You cannot serve both God and money." Paul is happy with what he has, and if he wants to save for something, he does so patiently without complaining until Mom or Dad let him know that he has enough money. Remember, he waited well over thirty years for Dad to get a new truck, so a few months is nothing to him!

Paul traditionally has expensive taste, so he finds himself waiting, more often than not, for an item on his wish list. He doesn't demand the latest technological gadgets, and he certainly doesn't feel the need to flaunt new possessions if he does get them. An example of this occurred recently when he asked Mom if he could have a flat screen television for his bedroom. They were grocery shopping at Wal-Mart when he pointed to the television displays, and then pointed to himself. He said, "Paul," followed by holding his hands up to his face and sleeping. He took the index finger of his right hand, and placed it in the middle of his left palm, moving his index finger back and forth in a half-circle, which is his sign language for money.

Mom explained that she would help him start saving money for a new television, but that he would have to wait until they saved enough. Several weeks later she took him back to Wal-Mart to make his purchase and he picked out one of the smallest television screens that still had high-quality features. He doesn't have to have the biggest or best of anything in life, but he is a smart shopper. I am humbled by the wisdom of his willingness to save money, along with his patience.

TAKE TIME TO ENJOY THE SIMPLE THINGS IN LIFE

One of Paul's favorite pastimes is to sit on his front porch swing and watch the world go by. Every year from spring until fall, Paul is on his porch swing a minimum of an hour each day, sometimes more. As long as there isn't lightning, he can be found out there. He loves to watch the neighboring farmers prepare and plant their fields. He looks forward to harvest, as if it were a beloved holiday. Through prayer, he even asks God to send rain when the land is dry, or to make the rain go away if there has been too much.

I am reminded of the Bible verse found in James 3:18, "Peacemakers who sow in peace raise a harvest of righteousness." With Paul's love of planting and harvesting fields to produce corn and beans, he also lives by planting and sowing righteousness through his actions.

Paul has an internal clock that knows instinctively when farmers should plant or harvest. This internal clock causes him to become agitated if he thinks the farmers are not moving fast enough to plant seeds or harvest their fields. He is very opinionated when it comes to beans and corn. When it is finally time to harvest, he will begin motioning scissor cutting with his fingers, simulating a combine cutting the crops, and repeatedly suggests that they should do the obvious—cut the corn and beans!

Another of Paul's favorite things is to enjoy a bottle of ice-cold Coca Cola. He will ask for a Coke on his birthday or Christmas, and it is worth a million dollars in his mind. How many of us in today's rushed society actually take the time to quietly enjoy a drink? When I do take the time to enjoy one, I notice that it really does taste better. It is much more satisfying and therefore I do not feel like I need another one immediately afterward.

Paul also loves to celebrate anything for any reason at all. We still have to have birthday parties for my oldest nieces and nephews who are in their twenties because Paul loves birthdays. Truth be told, I think what he loves most is the bounty of food from the pitch-in meals, but the birthday celebration takes a strong second place.

I have never heard him complain because he didn't want to disrupt his weekend plans and go to a birthday party. It is not an obligation that he is simply fulfilling; he takes time to enjoy the opportunity, the sparkle of the lit candles, the birthday cake for the birthday boy or girl, and blowing out the candles before they do! Consider the next birthday party you attend from Paul's point of view; you are lucky to have that person in your life and time spent together is hardly a sacrifice. Enjoy the moment.

Doctors' offices are often a weekly part of Paul's life; he has spent his fair share of time in many waiting rooms. Paul doesn't complain about how long he must wait to see the doctors, but instead uses the wait as an opportunity to greet others with a friendly smile. And, while he doesn't like missing a day of work, he enjoys the opportunity to take a trip to Indianapolis and eat at his lifelong favorite hamburger joint, White Castle. The fact that Mom and Dad selflessly take him to White Castle should earn them an extra star in Heaven, because White Castles and Paul's digestive system do not complement each other.

BE PROUD OF WHO YOU ARE

Paul is very comfortable being the person that he is. The doctors have encouraged Mom to help Paul lose weight over the years. The problem is, Santa Claus has a nice round belly, and Paul wants to be like Santa. When our oldest sister-in-law, Carla, became pregnant with their first child, Paul stopped talking to her because he did not like that her belly was bigger than his. He is proud of his belly, and this has proven to be the most difficult task for my parents to conquer. One embarrassing issue that I have experienced with Paul continues to occur when he sees an overweight person out in public and he thinks that he is complimenting them on their "fat belly." There are some things that he tries to say that are difficult for outsiders to understand, but unfortunately this is a topic where his communication is impeccable and they clearly get the message that he is talking about their waistline! "Do you know that your body is a temple of the Holy Spirit, who is in you, who you have received from God?" (1 Corinthians 6:19).

Take Time to Laugh—What a Gas!

Paul can make himself comfortable in almost any location, and I have never experienced him acting or pretending to be any different than his true self. The problem with this is that he thinks passing gas is funny, and he is really proud of the sonic blasts he has emitted over the years. He can clear out an entire room within seconds if he wants to, and he will continue to sit in the room quietly with a huge smile on his face.

To be honest, there have been times where Paul has mortified me with his public, gastric blasts, but one particular story is superior to all others. It was in 2007 and we were all in a hospital waiting room, praying desperately as a family for God to spare the life of my then, forty-two-year-old brother, Steve, who had just suffered a massive heart attack and stroke.

While Steve was in surgery, we joined together in the waiting room as a family, supporting each other. I had a very close relationship with Steve and could not stop crying; the intense fear of losing such a significant person in my life was more than unbearable at that moment. I was sitting next to Paul on a small couch in the waiting room. I knew my tears were upsetting him even more, so I moved to the couch across from him so I could turn my head and pray for God to quiet my fears.

As I prayed for Him to give me the strength to accept whatever the outcome of Steve's heart surgery might be, I noticed a much older lady being pushed in a wheel chair to the seat next to Paul. The elderly woman could not stand without assistance, and after her caretaker safely guided her into the seat, she left the waiting room for a few minutes. Paul stared at the elderly woman, looked around at us, and stared at the caretaker leaving the room.

I could see in Paul's eyes that he needed to be alone, and that he found the presence of the decrepit old woman to be annoyingly close. I was making matters worse with my inability to hold myself together. And, although I may have already been in a state of shock, the ensuing events played out before me in slow motion; I could see them coming, but had no time to respond. Paul loves to make people laugh and smile, and part of me knows that he wanted her to laugh, too.

Paul casually twisted his body around so that his back side was facing the lady, and lifted himself slightly off the seat. Before we could stop him, he passed gas. I can still hear it in my head today. The smell was unfortunately atrocious and there was not a thing we could do about it. I believe that he wanted to break the tension of the hospital waiting room, and make us and the others around, laugh. He succeeded. I must remind him, however, that the Bible does say "Whoever flatters their neighbor is spreading a net for his feet . . ." (Proverbs 29:5). He was reprimanded by Dad. And personally, I went from not being able to stop crying, to not being able to stop laughing. Paul was obviously "cutting" the tension in the room. His message, while rude and crude, was to use laughter to get through difficult moments in life.

IF YOU CAN'T BEAT THEM, JOIN THEM

By now it is understood that Paul loves eating and having a nice round belly. Mom is mindful of everything he eats, and she makes sure he walks or rides his bike daily. Instead of losing pounds, however, he continues to gain weight as food disappears mysteriously from the kitchen.

One evening my three children wanted to hang out with Paul and have a sleepover at my parents' house. A few hours after everyone went to bed, my daughter Arianna, heard noises coming from the kitchen. Fully expecting to see her Grandma in the kitchen, Arianna came upon Paul making a midnight snack. Arianna knew that he was supposed to be in bed and asked him if he should be making toast in the middle of the night. Paul looked at her and with a finger pressed to his lips he said, "Shhhh!" Next, he buttered a piece of toast for her, and then walked her back to her bed before he headed back upstairs to his.

The next morning when Mom was preparing breakfast she asked Arianna what she wanted to eat. Unfortunately for Paul, Arianna responded that she had buttered toast with Paul only a few hours before and wasn't hungry yet. At least Mom was able to find out where the missing food went! Paul loves his family and his food. "For where your treasure is, there your heart will be also . . ." (Matthew 6:21).

DON'T JUDGE OTHER PEOPLE

There are so many things that I love about Paul, but his ability to love everyone takes first place. He is a mentor in this area of my life and this ability to love is something that he has mastered better than anyone I know. Paul does not care if someone is rich or poor, black or white, gay or straight, blond-haired or black, gothic or punk, atheist or not; he will still shake your hand. He only sees the best in people and does not get hung up on rumor or trivialities. Even when people have disrespected Paul because they thought he was "stupid" or because he wasn't "normal," Paul still shakes their hand and smiles. A friend of mine once said after seeing Paul at an air show, "If the entire world treated each other like Paul treats people, it would be a much happier place." Hebrews 13:2 reminds us, "Do not forget to entertain strangers, for by so doing some people have entertained angels without knowing it."

Paul is a social genius, and he has been his entire life. He is not afraid or embarrassed to be himself around anyone, and most often has a warm smile and a genuine handshake waiting for anyone who walks by. Paul has an inner light that shines through his eyes. Luke 11:34 says, "Your eye is the lamp of your body. When your eyes are good, your whole body also is full of light. But when they are bad, your body also is full of darkness. See to it, then, that the light within you is not darkness."

GIVE BACK TO THE CHURCH AND COMMUNITY

The offering plate is passed around twice on Sunday mornings, and Paul places in it a dollar from his billfold with each passing. As much as Paul treasures his dollar bills, he understands the greater good in giving to God with an open, happy heart. If a collection jar sets out for a community fundraiser, Paul will draw out his billfold and make his contribution. He gives so much of what he has, but he expects nothing in return. I think of him when I read the verse "I tell you the truth, whatever you did for one of the least of these brothers of mine, you did for me" (Matthew 25:40).

SHOW GRATUITY

In the same way that he generously tithes his dollar bills on Sundays, Paul will not leave a restaurant without personally leaving a one-dollar tip for the waiter or waitress. It doesn't matter if we leave a twenty-dollar tip on the table, Paul will not leave until he has left his own gratuity. He includes an extra tip even if he has had terrible service! Paul understands giving and serving others without expecting anything in return. Mark 10:45 reminds us that "For even the Son of Man did not come to be served, but to serve, and to give his life as a ransom for many."

BE FUN TO BE AROUND

Paul is so much fun to be around. He sees the best in everyone and enjoys making others laugh. He rarely lets pain slow him down. Matthew 7:17 says that "every good tree bears good fruit, but a bad tree bears bad fruit." If this is so, then metaphorically Paul is a strong, bountiful tree. His arms are open wide, and he is ready to have fun wherever, whenever, and with whomever.

DON'T WORRY, BE HAPPY

I have to remind myself continuously to model Paul's sense of contentment. When he has to have a sinus surgery or some other complicated procedure done, he does not allow it to affect his day. He may be in a lot of pain, but he will not allow worry to take over. I think of how often I have lost sleep, worrying about things and allowing them to steal my joy. Paul lives his life according to the Bible verses "Therefore do not worry about tomorrow, for tomorrow will worry about itself. Each day has enough trouble of its own" (Matthew 6:34). It could be argued that because of his disability, Paul is not able to compute the ramifications of things. The point is valid. But in the end, he doesn't let worry strip him of his happiness, and we shouldn't either. For Matthew 6:27 reminds us, "Who of you by worrying can add a single hour to his life?"

Closing

I have always loved and treasured my parents, but their selflessness and devotion to Paul earns them a respect that I have for no one else. Because of their unconditional love and absolute commitment, Paul continues to bless this earth with his remarkable being. They, too, model unconditional love, respect, and a strong work ethic, and I am blessed as a result of it. Being Bear means loving others more than yourself, taking care of what you have, enjoying the simple things in life, not complaining, and praising God through prayer and actions, not just words. I know my life would have turned out differently had I not experienced life with my brother Paul. He continues to teach me life lessons, and most of all, he frequently reminds me to step back and enjoy all aspects of life. A smile and hug from him comfort my mind and soul. Paul is my hero.

THROUGH MY EYES

(The following is a poem that I wrote from Paul's perspective to Mom and Dad.)

What I see through my eyes is the purest love
without disguise.
I am not too old or filled with pride to say thanks
for standing by my side.
I live my life the best I can; it's just that I need your
helping hand.
When my lungs fill up, and I have no air, it makes
me calm because you're there.
Making sacrifices is your way, and because of this
I've lived many more days.

You never see me as a burden or pain but as your son with a voice and a name.

I know you can see the love in my eyes, but my brain lacks the words for me to describe

How much I love you and thank God, for I'm so glad

That I get to share such a journey with the best mom and dad!

One day I will see Jesus and to him I'll clearly say

Thanks for making me, me. I wouldn't want it any other way!

For I live my life with honesty, compassion, and love.

And I honor my personal Savior in Heaven above.

CHAPTER ELEVEN

An Interview with Bear
April 19th, 2012
Greencastle, Indiana

Joy: Bear, did you know that I am writing a book about you?

Paul: Yep.

Joy: What would you like me to tell people reading the book about you?

Paul: The airplane. (He is going to Florida soon.)

Joy: Who is your favorite person, me or Brian?

Paul: I want to call Santa Claus.

Joy: What do you love most about Christmas?

Paul: Have a merry, merry Christmas!

Joy: Where are you going on your next vacation?
Paul: On vacation? On an airplane.
Joy: Did you make a lot of money at work today?
Paul: Yep.
Joy: What do you want for your birthday?
Paul: A tape.

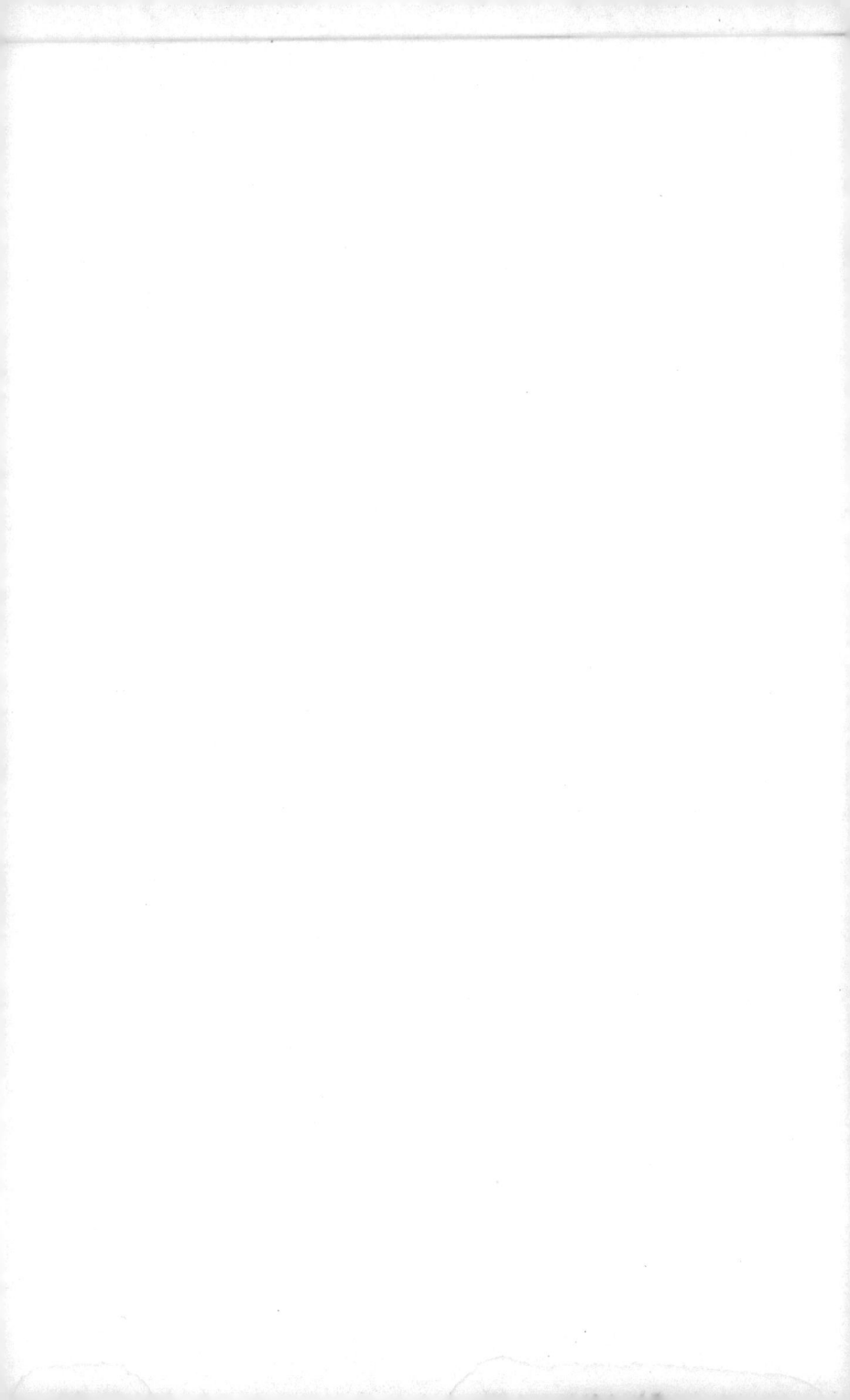

CPSIA information can be obtained at www.ICGtesting.com
Printed in the USA
LVOW120349291112

309298LV00002B/2/P